Matcha Tea

How this Super-Tea will
make you Unstoppable

Richard Foster Fletcher

CONTENTS

About the Authors

Richard Foster Fletcher and Suranjana Banerjee are writers at Teaologists.co.uk.

Teaologists.co.uk is a specialist importer and retailer of the highest quality Organic Ceremonial Grade Matcha Tea. Teaologists.co.uk is passionate about Matcha Tea and on a mission is to help as many people as possible to start their personal Daily Matcha Habit.

With so many mind, body and soul benefits, Teaologists believe that just one bowl or cup of Matcha each morning can change the world.

Teaologists.co.uk Ceremonial Grade Matcha tea is the very best available, it is 100% organic and sourced directly from carefully selected family owned Japanese Tea Plantations.

1 The History of Matcha Tea

Matcha tea has been produced and consumed in its modern form for many centuries. With an amazing 1,300 year history it precedes the renaissance artists, Copernicus and in fact all of our 'modern era'. Whilst Matcha is known as a Japanese tea, the original concept of grinding and drinking green tea leaves comes from China, where history shows this practice taking place as early as the eighth century.

In 960 AD, Chan (Zen) Buddhists in China adopted the practice of drinking Matcha. They had discovered that green tea could be pulverised into a pleasant drink that utilised the whole nutritional leaf. At this time, the tea was provided to the monks in solid chunks. This solidification of tea was necessary to transport the tea more easily and was achieved by steaming the leaves, then drying them and packing them into stiff moulds. The monks would break the cube apart and mash it using a pestle and mortar to obtain a fine powder. They would then whisk the fine powder into hot water and then drink slowly from a shallow bowl. The act of drinking tea this way held a special place in their lives. It is this act that would eventually evolve into the famous tea ceremony.

The Arrival

As time went by, the popularity of powdered tea

started to reduce and Matcha eventually lost the glory it once enjoyed among Chinese intellectuals. In China, Matcha was being replaced by other Chinese teas, especially *pu-her* as trends came and went. However, as consumption declined in China, Matcha was gaining more and more attention in Japan. The Zen monasteries of Japan had heard that drinking Matcha would help the monks to stay awake and alert during their long hours of meditation. History tells us that Matcha was consumed more like a tonic or medicine by these monks and therefore drunk relatively quickly in comparison to the tea ceremony practices of China.

We are fortunate to know the story of how Matcha was introduced to Japan. It was the year 1191 and a prominent monk named Eisai Myoan (1141-1215) planted the first green tea seeds in Japanese soil. Myoan was influential in society, and during the 1180s he travelled to China to learn and explore. Whilst there he discovered and quickly fell in love with Matcha and the Zen way of life. When he returned to Japan, he brought both the tea and the Zen teachings with him. The remainder of his life was spent devoted to teaching and writing about his two new discoveries. His two-volume *Kissa Yojouki (Book of Tea and Mulberries)* is one of the most seminal writings ever on Matcha tea.

The Rise

From the Zen monasteries, Matcha surprisingly,

perhaps, was not adopted immediately by the ruling class. Instead it gained popularity albeit slowly, among the general public as they found enjoyment in the rituals and social aspects of the tea ceremony. Eventually it found its way to the intellectual strata, and was adopted by the Samurai warriors around this time. The warriors, known as *Shogun*, realised the amazing benefits of Matcha. They drank Matcha before going to the battlefield, as it gave them sustained energy and improved their mental alertness. Matcha's popularity continued to grow in Japan through the end of the sixteenth century. As this new custom swept the nation, many rules quickly emerged for how Matcha tea must be taken.

Drinking and appreciating Matcha tea like an art form became a part of Japanese culture. Matcha was not unlike art forms such as flower arrangement, poetry or painting. Being comfortable in the act of preparing and consuming Matcha was considered prestigious, so much so that feudal lords would employ tea masters and collect tea paraphernalia to establish themselves as part of the elite society.

By the sixteenth century a prominent tea master by the name of Sen No Rikyū (1522 – 1591) was creating a name for himself. He was the tea master of choice for a number of the most powerful samurai warlords including Oda Nobunaga (1534 – 1582) who initiated the unification of Japan near the end of the Warring

States period. Rikyū dedicated his life to tea and with pioneered the transformation of the Matcha tea ceremony into a complex and choreographed ritual which featured several art forms including; architecture, lacquerware, ceramics, calligraphy, flower arrangement, painting, design, culinary arts and gardening. The Matcha tea ceremony is remarkable in how many varied forms of art are included.

For some time, whilst popular with the masses, Matcha was grown in limited quantities so that it was available to only the *Shogun* and the elite. This limiting could have been an effort to raise the price and exclusivity of the tea, or it may have been due to the cost and expertise required to create Matcha. Either way in 1738, a prominent tea-master Sohen Nagatani (1681 - 1778) invented a green tea preparation technique that he called "*uji*". Uji was originally kept very secretive as it was far more efficient than previous methods. Nagatini made a daring decision to share his knowledge with a group of farmers and this one act revolutionised forever the way Matcha was created and processed. This easier and cheaper processing made Matcha readily accessible for the 'common people' of Japan. The uji technique is still in practice today.

With the transformation of the Matcha cultivation, tea growers started applying better cultivation techniques and enriching their knowledge of these techniques.

This continual improvement process improved the quality of Matcha with every cultivation. Whilst Matcha was gaining mainstream popularity, the Zen Buddhists desired that the tea ceremony remain an occasion to celebrate the simple things in life and promote better meditation. The ceremony had its own aesthetic principles, called *sabi* and *wabi*. Sabi is a metaphor for the 'material' things in life and wabi has more to do with life's spiritual aspects. The noblemen believed that understanding emptiness was the best path to nirvana and that they should embrace all imperfection along the way.

With tea drinking becoming common practice among all societies in Japan, there emerged a philosophy that the tea ceremony was a unique experience that can never be replicated and thus should be cherished. This philosophy led to the creation of new forms of art and architecture, along with the development of what we now know as the 'way of tea'. The principles of the way of tea are purity, tranquillity, harmony and respect. These principles are still observed in Japanese tea ceremonies today.

The consumption of Matcha tea was at first limited to men, especially monks and influential men of society. Women were included much later, but today, women dominate the practice of tea ceremonies.

Present Day

For over 800 years, Matcha tea has held a very special place in the Japanese culture and lifestyle. Though all the benefits of Matcha were experienced by those who drank it in ancient times, modern scientific research can now explain how these benefits are derived and the positive implications for our modern lives. Nowadays people in countries far away from Japan are able to access Matcha. The popularity of this great green tea is now more widespread than ever. Matcha has gone beyond tea ceremonies and is enjoyed on its own as an enjoyable beverage, as a healthy drink and as a workout enhancing pre-drink in many countries. In Japan however, the tea ceremonies still remains an integral part of society.

As a company, teaologists.co.uk actively promotes the benefits of drinking one bowl or cup of Matcha tea every day as we share a vision that Matcha tea will be enjoyed by people all over the world and become an important part of each and every culture.

2 How to Make Matcha Tea

The modern preparation method of Matcha tea takes its elements from the ancient tea ceremonies. But nowadays with our busy lives, it is normal to make

Matcha quickly and efficiently without the ceremonial pomp and circumstance. So here are the modern-day instructions for making Matcha tea:

Ingredients:

- Matcha Tea
- Water

Tools You Need:

- Tea Bowl (Japanese Name: *Chawan*)
- Bamboo Whisk (Japanese Name: *Chasen*)
- Bamboo Spoon (Japanese Name: *Chashaku*)
- Sifter Or Sieve (Japanese Name: *Furui*)

Method:

First, you need to heat up the water, as Matcha tastes best when it's blended at near boiling point (ideal temperature of the water should be somewhere between 70°C to 80°C). Put the kettle on and let it sit for a few moments. Gather your tools. With the hot water, rinse the inside of your tea bowl to make sure the ideal heat is maintained. Then take 1 teaspoon or *Chashaku* of Matcha and sift it through a small sieve into the bowl. Do not force the tea through the sieve. Simply shake it through and gently apply pressure to the little leftover clumps to produce a fine powder in the bowl. Don't worry about perfection here, quality Matcha will always be a little clumpy.

You can make Matcha in two ways: *usucha* and *koicha*. Usucha is the light (thin) version of Matcha tea, whilst koicha refers to the thick version. Both are popular.

Take the water off the heat and pour it slowly into the bowl. Now take the whisk in one hand and use your other hand to hold the Matcha bowl steady. To make usucha, whisk the tea briskly for a few seconds in a "W" or "M" motion. Do not whisk in a circular motion as it doesn't blend the tea well in the water. That is to say, the tea can be lumpy if you use a circular whisking motion—but never with a "W" or "M" motion. When you can no longer see any lumps, a thick froth with lots of tiny bubbles on its surface should have formed, at this point stop whisking and drink the tea directly from the bowl.

To make koicha, whisk in a left-to-right and up-and-down motion. Also, add a 360-degree rotating motion to get a thick consistency. When you are about to touch the bowl's surface, slow down the whisking, as this will break the big bubbles on the surface.

Drink directly from the cup or bowl. This version of Matcha will not be frothy.

Additional Tips: Ideally you should use a sturdy bowl that is wide enough to accommodate the quick whisking in various different motions. Do not use a metal whisk. You can use a milk frother in lieu of a whisk but using a bamboo whisk is the best way to make Matcha.

Problems That You Can Encounter and How to Solve Them:

- Bitter taste. If the Matcha tastes bitter, the reason could be any of the following three: 1) the water was too hot, 2) the quantity of Matcha was more than what's recommended and 3) the tea wasn't whisked well. Matcha must be whisked well until a thick froth is achieved. If you can see breaks in the froth or large bubbles on the surface, that means the tea won't taste as good as it should.

- The tea doesn't froth well. This is a common occurrence when the Matcha is not whisked thoroughly, but it also happens when too much Matcha and/or too much water has been used. If this is encountered you should either increase the amount of tea or reduce the amount of water.

- Lumps in the Matcha. Lumps can show up if you don't sift the tea. Simply sift the tea before pouring water on it and the lumps will no longer affect your Matcha drinking experience.

3 Become Unstoppable with Matcha Tea

Bright green in colour and packed with health benefits, Matcha might be *the* health supplement you are looking for. In fact, it may be time to replace your regular green tea with Matcha. After all, Matcha is a superfood! One serving of Matcha has up to 137 times the disease-fighting polyphenols named *epigallocatechin gallate* (better known as EGCG), than one cup of green tea. This means that the goodness of 10 cups of green tea is in 1 cup of Matcha tea. Not only that, when you drink Matcha tea, you actually consume the whole tea leaf, contrary to other teas where you consume only a brew of its leaves.

Losing Weight

Matcha tea is, in fact, still a secret that a lot of people are still in the process of discovering. Think of it as a supercharged version of green tea that helps you lose weight naturally. If you've been looking to kick-start your weight-loss regime, drinking Matcha is a must. It will allow an exponential increase in the health benefits that come from your diet and exercise. It will actually boost your metabolism so that you burn more calories.

How Matcha helps with weight loss:

- Apart from speeding up your metabolism, Matcha also keeps your body from storing excess fat
- It suppresses your appetite naturally
- It gives your body a huge boost of antioxidants
- The huge amount of EGCG in Matcha tea reduces cholesterol in your body, inhibiting the risk of heart disease
- The same EGCG helps in treating diabetes and is reported to have a glucose-reducing impact. Basically, Matcha helps you control the insulin levels in your body, which in turn helps you control your appetite
- Matcha increases fat oxidation in your body, which helps your body use fat as a source of energy (meaning, the body burns fat instead of protein)
- Matcha contains catechins, which, according to a 2005 study in the *American Journal of Clinical Nutrition*, helps with weight loss. Catechins are associated with lower BMI and waist circumference. (*The study suggested that catechins alone cannot have an effect on reducing BMI and waist circumference)

- Some research has shown that EGCG may stop new fat cells from growing. (*Results in humans are yet to be confirmed through new studies).

Due to so many fat-reducing properties, Matcha is a great addition to any weight loss programme. Whether you have been hitting the gym for a while, are just starting your new health regime, or simply taking steps forward to a healthier lifestyle, Matcha tea is a force to be reckoned with.

However, Matcha is not a magic solution to all weight problems. When combined with a healthy diet and regular exercise, regular consumption of Matcha can lead to very positive results. It can also give your body a gentle stimulating effect much superior to that of steeped teas.

Looking and feeling younger.

Matcha is an anti-ageing miracle food. Research has shown that Matcha has anti-inflammatory and antibacterial properties, which help slow down the effects of ageing. In fact, the powdered green tea has such a wide range of age-delaying effects that it's difficult to sum them all up in a single book.

Below are some of the anti-ageing benefits of Matcha tea.

- Matcha fights age-related disorders such as dementia and Alzheimer's
- It has L-Theanine which helps to fight cardiovascular diseases
- The EGCGs in Matcha bind and stabilise transthyretin tetramer structures, which help the body combat Parkinson's disease and Huntington's disease
- Matcha has a positive impact on the bone density, bone recovery and bone structure of the body
- Regular consumption of Matcha for a long time decreases the fat deposits in the hippocampus, which reduces the age-induced decline of memory
- The polyphenols in Matcha tea help decrease the ultraviolet damage to the retina. This means that Matcha can help fight age-induced vision disorders like macular degeneration too
- Matcha tea helps the body to combat osteoporosis
- Regular application of Matcha extracts on the skin helps the skin's elasticity and viscosity
- The antioxidants in this green tea powder boost the oxygen supply to the heart
- Regular consumption of Matcha prevents diminishing spatial feeling, which is an effect of ageing
- The metabolites in Matcha have a positive impact on amino acids and the EGCG in

Matcha decreases the production of lipofuscin in the body. Lipofuscin refers to fine granular pigments that build up in the kidney, adrenals, liver, retina, heart muscle, nerve cells, and ganglion cells. These are the body's "wear and tear" pigments. Matcha slows down the build-up and therefore slows down the effects of ageing on the body

- The EGCGs in Matcha provide protection to the nerve cells

For a long, long time, Matcha has been known as the "the elixir of immortality" among the Chinese. It has catechin polyphenols, compounds that make it an anti-ageing superfood. Its anti-inflammatory properties promote skin health. The green tea powder can also be used in skin treatments to protect against blemishes. It's very easy to use as well. All you need to do is mix a small amount of Matcha with water to make a paste and apply it on your face and leave it for about 20-25 minutes. When you wash it off, you will have baby soft skin.

If you want to reap all the anti-ageing benefits of Matcha, make sure you drink 2-3 cups a day on a regular basis.

Bonus Tip: Make a flawless-skin mask right at home by mixing 1 tablespoon of culinary grade Matcha with yoghurt and honey. Use only a little bit of honey (otherwise the mask will be sticky).

Having more energy

L-Theanine counteracts the overstimulation of adrenaline or cortisol caused by caffeine intake. This can offer lasting energy, without the crashes and dips of coffee and energy drinks. The catechins in Matcha regulate caffeine and provide a much steadier energy boost than any energy drink, coffee, or black tea. Drinking Matcha tea regularly gives a boost to concentration and alertness and promotes a sense of well-being, thanks to the high levels of the L-Theanine amino acid.

The energy benefits of Matcha tea:

- Increased Energy: When you drink Matcha on a regular basis you feel more energetic than before. You stay energetic longer but never feel overstimulated. The L-Theanine amino acid in Matcha tea promotes clarity of mind and calmness.

- Less Fatigue: The habit of a daily Matcha intake can make you feel less tired. It effectively balances your blood sugar levels so that you don't feel a sudden drop in your productivity. In fact, your physical endurance is increased by up to 24% with regular intake of Matcha tea.

- Increased Concentration: For centuries, Matcha tea has been used to improve concentration. Zen monks consumed Matcha to stay focused during their long hours of meditation and Samurai drank it to boost their alertness and attention before going into battle. The marked increase in energy that Matcha provides comes from its L-Theanine, which also helps cope with stress and lifts the mood.

- Keeping Cravings in Check: Since Matcha releases energy slowly in the bloodstream, this keeps the blood sugar levels balanced. In turn, you don't crave a mid-afternoon chocolate bar or something to snack on in the evening. It just doesn't happen.

- Sense of Well-Being: Matcha gives you a feeling of well-being that stays with you. You feel less stressed, more positive and calmer.

- Better, Deeper Sleep: We all know how important a good night's sleep is. The high levels of L-Theanine in Matcha keep you more relaxed, which leads to a good night's sleep. Sleep patterns improve and you wake up feeling absolutely fresh and energised.

A study in the *American Journal of Clinical Nutrition* showed that there are unique thermogenic properties in Matcha, which boost the body's thermogenesis—the rate at which the body burns calories—from 10% to 40%. This means Matcha helps your body burn up to four times more calories and fat.

How Matcha Bypasses the Jittery Rush of Coffee:

One serving of Matcha contains 30-40 mg of caffeine, whilst one cup of coffee contains 200 mg of caffeine. Apart from having considerably less caffeine, there is a substantial amount of antioxidants in Matcha, which promote calmness. Because of minimal caffeine content, high levels of antioxidants and the fact that Matcha releases energy into the bloodstream very slowly, you get up to 6 hours of added energy without the jitteriness of coffee.

Bonus Tip: Even though there is much less caffeine in Matcha than in coffee, you should still limit your daily intake of this green tea. Three cups a day is ideal. Try taking it 30 minutes before you start your workout.

Illness Recovery

When you are unwell, it is especially important to maintain a healthy diet and lifestyle to help your body recover fast. Drinking Matcha tea during sickness is reported to yield speedy recovery, depending on your illness. For centuries, Matcha has been a remedy for many illnesses. Modern research shows that Matcha does have a lot of anti-infective and anti-inflammatory properties that offer considerable health benefits.

Matcha tea is a natural source of:

- L-Theanine: An amino acid that works wonders, from promoting a sense of well-being to boosting mental alertness and reducing stress.
- Vitamin C.
- Antioxidants: There is 100 times more antioxidants in one cup of Matcha than in one cup of green tea. The antioxidants promote the oxygen supply to your heart.
- Soluble and insoluble fibers.

Matcha tea is produced using a very natural technique—by grinding whole tea leaves. Nothing is added to it, and nothing is taken away. It's as pure as they come. So, when you drink Matcha tea you get nothing but the goodness of whole tea leaves, which are rich in the aforementioned properties, along with:

- Caffeine: Caffeine is released slowly into the bloodstream and doesn't make you feel the jittery rush you feel after drinking coffee.

- Anti-inflammatory properties: The EGCG or epigallocatechin-3-gallate in Matcha tea helps suppress inflammation and prevent swelling, fever, pain and general discomfort. *

- Anti-infective properties: According to research published in the December 2011 issue of *Hepatology*, EGCG inhibits the hepatitis C virus from infecting cultured liver cells. This suggests that it could help people who are infected by the virus. That means, those who are suffering from an illness caused by a pathogen, can benefit from the goodness of EGCG. *

In addition to all these, the EGCG in Matcha can also neutralise free radicals in your body. Free radicals can wreak havoc in the DNA structure and the cellular membranes, and increase your chances of contracting a chronic illness.

*Yet to be confirmed through clinical studies.

Protection against Cancer

Matcha decreases the risk of cancer in the body. The green tea is packed with cancer-fighting antioxidants known as catechins which slow down the growth of tumours in the pancreas, liver, stomach, intestines, bladder, and even the brain, without having any apoptotic effect on the healthy cells. They also break the molecular link between infection and cancer.

Each serving of Matcha comes with a heavy dose of EGCG. According to researchers, EGCG can do the following:

- Kill cancerous cells
- Stop the spread of breast cancer, lung cancer, prostate cancer, colon cancer, cancer of the oesophagus
- Influence medication
- Scavenge free radicals in the body, thereby preventing DNA damage

EGCG makes up for about 60% of all the catechins in Matcha. According to emerging clinical studies, EGCG helps rid the body of free radicals that enter the body through radiation, pollution, and chemicals. These all can potentially damage cells.

Drinking Matcha tea on a regular basis can have a significant impact on reducing the risk of developing many types of cancer. The National Cancer Institute (NCI) in the USA suggests that the catechins found in Matcha green tea are so powerful that they have the ability to prevent cancer.

Research shows that these catechins can even improve the function of the entire immune system of the body. They also release quinone reductase and S-transferase, detoxification enzymes which are known to hinder tumour growth.

So it's safe to say that Matcha is a natural cancer fighter.

Bonus tip: If you are looking to benefit from a healthy diet, include a daily intake of 3 cups of Matcha tea.

Detoxing

Detoxification is an ancient process to cleanse the body and to purge it of toxins and waste matter. The process is a natural one. It rids the body of harmful elements through the lungs, skin, kidneys and bowels. Depending on the body structure, detoxification can help with weight loss.

Detoxification improves overall health and promotes well-being. It provides a boost to energy levels, improves immunity, decreases bloating, increases stamina, keeps skin healthy, and promotes deeper sleep.

Chlorophyll is a significant natural detoxifier and Matcha has an ample amount of chlorophyll in it, thanks to the shade-growing process which skyrockets the production of chlorophyll in the Matcha leaves. With Matcha, you drink the whole leaves and you get all the nourishment that those shade-grown, chlorophyll-rich leaves have to offer.

How detoxing with Matcha Helps You:

You benefit from the following when you detox with Matcha tea:

- Reduced risk of heart disease because Matcha lowers bad (LDL) cholesterol
- Reduced risk of cancer as Matcha is packed with catechins—antioxidants that remove free radicals in your body
- Increased thermogenesis, which is the body's ability to burn fats. Consuming Matcha tea can increase your body's thermogenesis from 8–10% to 35–43%
- Better neurological health: Matcha has lots of L-Theanine, an amino acid, which can boost cognitive health
- Improved oxygenation: Chlorophyll spreads oxygen around the body, which helps improve the process of oxygenation and cleanses the blood
- A balanced level of alkaline in your blood and tissues
- Removal of toxins from colon walls

Chlorophyll is so powerful that it can detox even heavy metals. It has adhesive cellulose in its cellular walls which stick to the metals and carry them out of the body as waste.

Loaded with magnesium, chlorophyll gives your body an energy boost. Magnesium is hard to find in daily diets these days due to heavy-food processing.

Bonus tip: You can incorporate Matcha in your daily diet in various ways. But the best one is the most traditional one. Whisk a bowl of Matcha every morning and drink straight from the bowl. It's a nutrient-rich way to start your day.

Calmness

For well over 800 years, Buddhist monks have been drinking Matcha tea to maintain focus and alertness during their long meditation sessions. Even Japanese samurai used to drink Matcha to stay calm and peaceful in their lives that were full of violence. Clearly, Matcha has calming properties, the source of which is—you guessed it—L-Theanine. This amino acid is the magic ingredient that reduces stress levels and boosts calmness and concentration.

To help you keep calm, we recommend daily cups of Matcha tea. It relaxes your mind and body and it works fast. You feel relaxed soon after drinking Matcha. The greener the Matcha, the higher the chlorophyll content and the more the relaxing effect.

Simply replace your morning coffee with a bowl of Matcha and reap these benefits:

- L-Theanine helps boost the alpha brain waves, which along with relieving you of stress and anxiety, also increases your concentration
- You get the goodness of vitamins A, B1, B2, B6, C, E and K

- You also benefit from minerals, such as magnesium, iron, potassium, phosphorus, and zinc
- Your blood pressure is lowered
- Your heart rate is calmed
- Your blood sugar levels are regulated, which means you don't experience energy dips that come with drinking coffee
- Unlike antidepressants, there are no side effects to drinking Matcha on a regular basis

So much calmness and yet you don't feel drowsy, that's the magic of Matcha. It offers tranquillity without drowsiness. So, no afternoon slumps to worry about!

4 The Different Types of Matcha

Matcha is different from almost all other teas in the world, in that it comes in powder form. It is made differently as well. There is no steeping of tea leaves in water. Instead, you have to brew the entire leaves (which are in powdered form) into the water and whisk it to a perfect broth.

When it comes to the best, most genuine Matcha tea, one name comes to mind: *gyokuro*. It's the most famous Japanese tea. Every year gyokuro plants are kept shaded for 20 days in early May to slow down the growth, boost the production of L-Theanine and mainly to bring that signature deep green colour.

Trivia: L-Theanine sweetens Matcha tea.

After those 20 days, the cover is removed and the larger buds are plucked to make *tencha*, which is basically the raw material for Matcha. To make tencha, the leaves are steamed (not rolled), then the veins and stalks are removed from them.

When powdered, green tea can stay fresh for a limited period of time, (15 days in the summer and 30 days in the winter). That's why the tencha leaves are stored until there is need for them to be finely stone-grounded into Matcha. Right after the stone-grinding, the tea (now Matcha) is packaged into airtight packaging and shipped.

So, there are 3 stages of Matcha green tea: gyokuro, tencha and Matcha.

How to Differentiate High-Quality Matcha from Low-Quality Matcha.

There are two main differences between high-quality

Matcha and low-quality Matcha. High-quality Matcha has a bit of astringency in it due to the concentrated level of L-Theanine. That's why it has a sweet and smooth taste. On the other hand, low-quality Matcha (or should we say powdered green tea?) has little to no L-Theanine, which makes it taste flat and rough.

High-quality Matcha is ground into a fine powder with the help of granite grinding wheels which move very slowly. There is the least friction in this process and that prevents the leaves from "burning," thus saving their chlorophyll content. But the grinding process of low-quality Matcha involves a lot of friction which gives the tea a yellowish brown colour and spoils its taste.

Grades

Three grades of Matcha are available: ceremonial grade, premium grade and culinary or cooking grade.

Ceremonial Grade

Ceremonial grade Matcha is the best. Its name derives from—you guessed it—Japanese tea ceremonies. Though it is hard to come by anywhere outside Japan, some companies are dedicated to building sustainable relationships with Japanese Tea Farmers to source and import the very best Matcha. Teaologists.co.uk are proud to be amongst this small number.

Due to its naturally sweet taste, ceremonial grade

Matcha is meant to be consumed without adding any sweetener to it. It must be blended with hot water in order for its delicate flavour to be "felt." It has a fresh, mildly grassy aroma and an extremely fine texture. The recommended amount to be used is half a teaspoon.

Premium Grade

Premium grade is the more "everyday use" Matcha. It's also a fine quality Matcha and is very popular, however the lower grade quality means a reduction in nutritional benefit and a sharper more bitter taste.

Culinary Grade

Culinary grade or cooking grade Matcha is, as the name suggests, used mainly in cooking, baking and in making flavoured beverages. It's a cheaper cousin of the above two grades and caters to a variety of uses. In order to stand out as a flavour, it needs a stronger "feel" and is therefore added to older tea leaves to get that strength. Culinary grade Matcha is used in ice creams, cakes, smoothies, chocolates, lattes, and so on

The flavour profile of culinary grade Matcha is bitter, astringent-like. That's why it must be mixed with other elements, such as milk, sugar, cream etc., to bring about a more appealing taste. Though less bright green than ceremonial and premium grade, it still has a nice emerald hue and feels soft and smooth to the touch. It has some of the fresh, grassy aroma of ceremonial Matcha as well. We recommend using 1 or 2 tablespoons of culinary grade Matcha. But if you prefer a stronger taste of tea, you can add more.

Trivia:

- Ceremonial grade Matcha will always be vividly green. If it's a yellowish green Matcha, it's not genuine ceremonial grade
- Culinary grade Matcha is supposed to be used as an ingredient. But a good quality culinary Matcha can still make you a nice cup of tea
- If culinary Matcha feels rough to the touch, it's an inferior quality culinary Matcha or it is probably way past its prime
- Many people are of the opinion that since culinary grade Matcha costs less than other grades, it's an inferior quality. But that's not really the case. It's a different grade

Types

Matcha is available in two types: *koicha* and *usucha*. Koicha refers to the thick variety of Matcha tea and usucha refers to the thin kind.

Koicha is brewed only in Japanese tea ceremonies whilst Usucha is the "everyday" variety.

The flavour profile of koicha is sweet and mellow due to the small amount of water used.

Usucha has a less sweet, thinner flavour profile, which makes it very frothy.

5 Ways to Drink Matcha

It's easy to get your daily dose of Matcha tea. In fact, it's easier than you think. You probably know the traditional way to drink Matcha—by whisking it in hot water in a bowl. Although that's the most popular way to drink it, there are other ways such as:

- Making Matcha latte
- Making Matcha lemonade
- Making Matcha smoothie

Thanks to the fact that it comes in a powdered form, Matcha tea is highly versatile. You can actually add it to any beverage you want. Even use it as a garnish.

We at Teaologists.co.uk have created the perfect Matcha beverage recipes which are simple enough to make on a workday and healthy enough to give you all the goodness of this emerald miracle.

Tip: You can replace coconut milk with dairy milk or soy milk, whichever you prefer.

Here's our guide to make Matcha tea the traditional way: bit.ly/trad-matcha

Too busy to buy the Matcha-making tools? No worries. There are alternative ways to brew Matcha at home. **Check out our guide to make Matcha without the tools**: bit.ly/notools

As long as you are getting your 1/2 a teaspoon of Matcha a day, you're all set.

How to Make Matcha Shots:

You need:

- A fruit juice of your choice
- Water or milk (hot or cold, whichever you like)
- Matcha tea, ½ teaspoon
- A shot glass

Pour the fruit juice into the shot glass. Add the Matcha and water/milk, whisk it with and drink it! You don't *have* to whisk it with a bamboo whisk, whilst this is the ideal option, a hand blender or milk frother will do just as well.

6 Matcha vs. Green Tea vs. Coffee

Caffeine

Whilst Matcha is rarely marketed as an energy drink, it certainly is one The caffeine content found in Match is much lower than that of coffee (about 25mg in one cup), but you have to keep in mind that the caffeine in it is different from that found in coffee.

- The caffeine in coffee gives the body a blast of energy which crashes after a while because it's released into the bloodstream too quickly. However, the caffeine in Matcha gives the body a stable boost of energy. The energy is released slowly into the bloodstream, resulting in an energy boost that stays for up to 6 hours. Even after that, it doesn't bring the feeling of exhaustion that coffee does.
- Coffee skyrockets adrenaline and insulin levels, creating jitteriness, anxiety and in some people, an insane hunger cramp. Matcha does no such thing. It promotes energy along with calmness and alertness, so that there are no energy ups and downs. Also, it satiates

hunger, eliminating the need for frequent snacks.

- Although it varies according to the brand and type, green tea has approximately 10-25 mg. of caffeine per 1 gram. However, the caffeine content in green tea also depends on the brewing time as well. The longer the brew, the more the caffeine content. Regular green tea does not release energy into the bloodstream as slowly as Matcha. So, the energy you get from consuming regular green tea is still less than what you get from Matcha, despite the fact that green tea itself is very healthy.

Antioxidants

- Matcha is loaded with antioxidants, especially catechins and epigallocatechin gallate (EGCG), which offer so many health benefits. These antioxidants combat free radicals in the body. If free radicals are allowed to build up over time, they can lead to chronic diseases and disorders.
- Coffee contains a fair amount of antioxidants as well, which promote energy, improve mood and help reduce the risk of many diseases. Coffee also causes jitteriness, which always comes with an impending crash. Not only that, drinking more than 2 cups of coffee a day can increase blood pressure and heart rate.

- Green tea contains lots of antioxidants, too, but not as many as Matcha. To put it into perspective, one bowl of Matcha tea contains the same amount of antioxidants as 10 cups of green tea.

Addictiveness

- Coffee is addictive. Due to the high amount of caffeine in it, coffee gives quick adrenaline spikes which are followed by sudden crashes. These crashes make one want to have more coffee to feel energetic again. The cycle goes on until an addiction can form.
- Green tea is not addictive. However, the caffeine in green tea is not released into the body as slowly as Matcha, so it could make you feel less satiated.
- Matcha is not addictive *at all*. Matcha bonds with other nutrients and takes time to do so. Due to the fact that there is only a little amount of caffeine in Matcha and even that is released over a long period time, Matcha does not lead to any crash, or a craving to have more.

7 How to Build a Matcha Habit

Human beings are creatures of habit. We are so committed to our habits that a study at Duke University suggested that habits account for about 40% of our behaviours.

As with every other habit, maintaining a healthy lifestyle and diet requires focus, commitment and determination. A good deal of understanding is required too. You have to understand what you can do and what you cannot. This is where you have to be completely honest with yourself. You must eliminate the "oh come on, I can't do this" moments at the first slip-up. That being said, let's delve into the ways you can train your body and mind to develop the habit of drinking something as healthy as Matcha tea on a regular basis.

You Need to Have a Clear Idea about Your Goal

What are you trying to achieve through this habit? That's the first question you should ask yourself. Is it just weight loss or an overall healthy body and mind that you seek? Or is it just because some friend recommended Matcha to you? When you have an honest answer from yourself, you'll know you've taken the first step to building one of the healthiest habits in the world.

Start Small

If you are not used to drinking Matcha, you can't just start drinking 3 bowls a day of all a sudden. Start with 1 bowl a day. That's easy enough and doesn't take much effort either. Give yourself time to adjust to the new habit. Since we are all creatures of habit, it won't take much time. Matcha is so good that it's hard to resist drinking it more than once a day.

Eliminate Too Many Options

Matcha is not the only healthy beverage out there. There are plenty others. But Matcha is far ahead of other healthy beverages in terms of its health benefits. So, try to pare down your decisions. You can't drink every healthy drink out there, and that's ok. Do you know why? Because you don't have to. Matcha is a superfood. It will give you all the health benefits you need.

Begin Early

Healthy habits, such as exercising or drinking Matcha, yield even better results if observed in the early morning. Whisk yourself a bowl first thing in the morning and you will enjoy its benefits all day.

Use a Trigger

A trigger is something that makes you connect one activity with another, like a chain reaction. For instance, many people feel like having a smoke after lunch or dinner. The meal, in this case, is the trigger to their smoking habit. If you are committed to developing a good habit, such as drinking Matcha, associate a trigger with it, such as laying out the tools to make Matcha in your kitchen at night, so that the next morning when you walk in there, those are the first things you see. But as mentioned above, Matcha is so good that it doesn't take this type of effort to build the habit of drinking it.

Document Your Progress

As you progress on your path to greater health, make sure to document the milestones. For every few pounds that you lose, you could write a diary entry. This will keep you focused and help you take notice of other health benefits you are enjoying because of the simple habit of drinking Matcha tea every day. Be very specific. The more specific you are, the better the next outcome will be and you will achieve your goal of a healthy lifestyle sooner than you think.

Finally, it's important to thank yourself for developing this wonderful habit. When you achieve your objective, thank yourself and make a promise to yourself to never quit this great habit.

8 Four Seasons Matcha Recipes

Seasons come and seasons go and there are Matcha recipes to enjoy whatever the weather. To impress your taste buds all throughout the year, here are some great Matcha recipes. We guarantee that you will adore these lovely dishes.

Summer

ICED MATCHA (GREEN TEA) WATERMELON

When watermelon and Matcha team up, cool things happen. They are like two best friends. They blend so very perfectly with each other. So here's a recipe for an iced Matcha watermelon drink. And here's the inside scoop: The colour of this drink is bright red and green! It comes in a stacked layer form, which looks so tempting!

The best thing about this drink is that there's no need to add sugar, as the natural sugar in the watermelon makes it sweet enough.

Let's do it.

Ingredients

Watermelon, seeded and cubed, around 2 cups

Water, half a cup

Teaologists organic culinary grade Matcha tea, 1 teaspoon

Ice cubes

Small watermelon wedges (for garnishing)

How to Make

Whisk the Matcha in the traditional method in a bowl using COLD water. Put the watermelon in the blender and make a smooth puree. Fill two glasses (the kind you use for "on the rocks" drinks) with ice cubes and pour the watermelon puree on them, followed by the Matcha. Slit the watermelon wedges a little and place them on the edges of the glasses as garnishing.

Serves 2.

Why You Shouldn't Use Ceremonial Grade Matcha When Cooking or Blending

Quality ceremonial Matcha has a very subtle taste, which can get lost in the process of blending with other flavours.

MATCHA YOGHURT

This is an excellent breakfast packed with nutritional value and it tastes amazing. The nutritional benefits of yoghurt are countless. It nourishes the immune system, and Greek yoghurt is high in protein content, which means that a little bit of it is enough to make you feel full.

Stress comes with a busy schedule, and with stress comes exhaustion. That's where this breakfast recipe comes in. It's super-easy to make and customise. If you are not in the mood to sit and eat, you can put this into a blender and turn it into a smoothie. You can add berries, slices of orange, walnuts, almonds—whatever topping you prefer. The result is a delicious, filling and healthy breakfast that will keep you energised till lunch time.

If you are adding Matcha in food for the first time, bear in mind that Matcha is not soluble like flavoured powdered black teas. So after you whisk it, just give it a nice, quick swirl with a spoon. That will be enough to evenly blend Matcha with the rest of the ingredients.

Without further ado, let's make some Matcha yoghurt.

Makes 1 breakfast bowl of yoghurt.

Ingredients

Yoghurt of your choice, 2/3 – ¾ cup (150-200ml)

Teaologists organic culinary grade Matcha, 1 tsp

Orange, 1 peeled and sliced

Maple syrup or honey to taste

Chopped almonds and walnuts, grated apple, seasonal berries.

How to Make

Sprinkle 1 teaspoon of Matcha over it. Add honey or maple syrup and whisk vigorously until it turns into a smooth paste-like mixture. Pour the mixture into a breakfast bowl and top with fruit, nuts and the sliced orange. Eat straight away.

Autumn

Matcha Goji Granola

Two superfoods unite to make a powerhouse of a food.

This granola will look uber-colourful! You can have it as breakfast or as a trail-mix that on your way to work. It oozes freshness and has a beautiful sweet taste.

Ingredients

Quinoa, 100 grams, cooked

Buckwheat groats, 150 grams (must be soaked overnight)

Sunflower seeds, 50 grams (soaked overnight)

Pumpkin seeds, 50 grams (also soaked overnight)

Goji berries, 50 grams

Coconut oil, 60 ml

Teaologists Organic Culinary Grade Matcha, 2 tablespoons

Chia seeds, 3 tablespoons

Sea salt, ¼ teaspoon

Maple syrup, to taste

Vanilla powder, 1 teaspoon

Shredded coconut, 3 tablespoons

How to Make

Pre-heat the oven to 165°C. Line a baking tray with baking paper. Rinse all the seeds well. Rinse the buckwheat as well. Add them to a bowl, along with the cooked quinoa, coconut oil, chia seeds, vanilla, maple syrup, and salt. Mix them. Make sure that the quinoa and buckwheat get a nice coating of the other ingredients on them. Now add 1 tablespoon of Matcha and the other ingredients except the goji berries. Mix well and pour the mixture on the baking tray. Spread it evenly onto the tray with the back of a spatula. Keep it outside the oven for 5 minutes. This will make everything bind with the chia seeds.

Put the tray in the oven and bake the mixture for 20 minutes. Make sure to rotate the baking tray so that the baking is even. Lower the temperature to 120°C and bake the mixture again for 30 minutes. Then, take out the tray, turn the mixture with a spatula and place the tray back inside. This time, bake for 15 minutes. Turn off the oven and allow the mix to sit inside for 30 minutes. Now bring it out from the oven and let it cool.

When it has cooled, add the second tablespoon of Matcha. Put in the goji berries and store it in an airtight container. You can have it over a period of several days with coconut yoghurt and nut milk.

Serves 4-6 to people.

Matcha Courgette Cake

Ingredients:

<u>The Courgette Cake:</u>

Courgette, 200 g

Honey, 50 g

Eggs, 3

Greek yoghurt, 200 g

Milled flaxseed and oat bran, 200 g

Cocoa powder, 50 g

Baking powder, 1 teaspoon

Bicarbonate of soda, 1 teaspoon

Splenda (or your choice of sweetener), 1 tablespoon

<u>The Matcha Filling:</u>

Teaologists Organic Culinary Grade Matcha, 1 tablespoon

Greek yoghurt, 200 g

Lime zest, ½

Splenda - 2 tablespoons

<u>The Chocolate Filling:</u>

Dark chocolate, – 60 g

Lime zest, ½

Avocado, 1

How to Make

Pre-heat the oven to 180°C.

Grate 200 g of Courgette in a bowl, add Greek yoghurt, honey and eggs. Mix well. Take another bowl, pour the baking powder, cocoa powder, Splenda, milled flaxseed and oat bran, and bicarbonate of soda. Mix them. Mix the contents of both bowls and line your baking tray with baking paper. Pour the mix and spread evenly with the back of a spoon. Bake it for 25 minutes. Then remove the tray from the oven and insert a knife into the middle of the cake. When you take the knife out, if you see traces of the cake on the blade, put the tray back in the oven and bake for a few minutes. Repeat the process until there's no cake residue on the knife.

Now it's time to make the Matcha filling. Combine all the ingredients of the filling and keep it the mixture in the fridge until the cake is fully baked.

Now the chocolate filling.

Put the dark chocolate in a heat-proof bowl and place the bowl over a pan of simmering water. Let the chocolate melt. 'Mash the flesh of the avocado and add to the melted chocolate along with the lime zest.

Blend until the texture is smooth and well mixed. Take a small bowl and line it with cling film. When the cake has cooled, cut it into slices and line the base and sides of the bowl. Take the Matcha filling and spread over all the cake in the bowl. Fill the centre with the chocolate avocado mixture. Top with the remainder of the cake. Seal with cling film and store in the fridge for 2 hours until ready to serve.

Winter

CREAMY MATCHA SOUP [VEGAN]

Who doesn't love simple recipes? And if those recipes are packed with proteins and antioxidants and yet come with few calories despite being extremely filling, then hey, they are nothing short of gems, right? So we've heard. We present you with one such gem of a recipe here. It's called creamy Matcha soup. You'll love it on a wintry night

Serves 4.

Ingredients

Potato, 1 medium, peeled and chopped

Onion, 1 medium, chopped

Teaologists organic culinary grade Matcha, 2 teaspoons

Garlic cloves, 4 minced

Ground black pepper, a pinch

Cayenne pepper, a pinch

Coriander - 1 cup of freshly chopped leaves

Coconut milk, 400 ml

Fresh kale, 5 full cups

Vegetable stock 4 cups (make sure it's low in sodium content)

How to Make

Heat a medium-sized pan and sauté the potato and onion in a little bit of vegetable stock (don't use the entire cup). Let it cook for about 8 minutes, stir occasionally and add water if required. Make sure the vegetables don't stick. Add the garlic, black pepper and cayenne, and sauté again for about 2 minutes. Add the kale and let it cook for a few minutes, then pour the rest of the vegetable stock, bring the soup to a boil and then turn the heat down to let it simmer. Cover the pan and let it cook for about half an hour. Add Matcha and Coriander stir gently and then let it cool for a while. Then pour it into a blender to make a silky smooth soup. After it's done, pour it back on a pot and add the coconut milk. Turn up the heat and let the heat distribute throughout the soup. Pour the soup in 4 bowls and serve hot.

MATCHA AND PISTACHIO CHOCOLATE TRUFFLES

How does a combination of antioxidant-rich Matcha, heart-healthy pistachios and glorious dark chocolate sound? "Out of this world!" we say. So let's tell you how to make Matcha and pistachio chocolate truffles.

Ingredients

Premium dark chocolate chips, 3 cups

Double cream, half a cup (doesn't have to be refrigerated; room temperature cream will do)

Pistachios, 1/3 cup, must be shelled and pulsed finely

Teaologists organic culinary Matcha, 1 tablespoon and 1 teaspoon for dusting

How to Make

Bring 2 to 3 cups of water to a simmer in a large saucepan. Place a stainless steel bowl or heatproof glass bowl over the saucepan. Add double cream, tablespoon of Matcha tea and chocolate chips to the bowl and stir well to let the chocolate melt and mix with the cream. Line the inside of a shallow bowl with greaseproof paper. Remove the bowl from the heat and pour the mixture into the bowl. Let it come down to room temperature. Then keep it in the fridge for about one a half hours. It will solidify.

After 1.5 hours, take it out from the fridge, scoop out the mix using a melon baller (a small one) and mold it into 1-inch balls. For those who don't have a melon baller, simply scoop the mix out with your hands.

Add the pistachios to a small bowl and roll the truffles in the ground pistachios, pressing them in well, then dust with sieved Matcha. Store in the fridge till needed.

Spring

MATCHA GREEN TEA COCONUT FLAN [VEGAN, GLUTEN-FREE]

An infusion of Matcha and coconut? When you are thinking of celebrating spring by making something super-amazing but don't have a lot of time to cook, consider this Matcha coconut flan.

INGREDIENTS

For the Crust:

Dried coconut, 3/4 cup, finely shredded

Flaxseed, half a cup, ground

Pitted dates, 1 cup

Buckwheat groats, 3/4 cup sprouted and dehydrated

Sea salt, ¼ teaspoon

For the Filling and Topping:

Fresh coconut meat, 4 cups (in case coconut meat is unavailable, the same amount of cashew can be used, but it has to be soaked for 4 hours)

Teaologists organic culinary grade Matcha, 1 tablespoon

Fresh coconut water, half a cup

Pure vanilla extract and vanilla bean seeds, half a tablespoon

Dried coconut flakes, 1 cup

Sea salt, 1/4 teaspoon

Raw coconut nectar, 1/4 cup and 2 tablespoons (you can replace it with your preferred liquid sweetener)

Melted raw coconut butter, 2/3 cup and 2 tablespoons

Some more coconut flakes and Matcha for garnishing

How to Make

Finely chop all the crust ingredients in a food processor and squeeze them. If they don't hold together, add some more dates to the mix. Take a 6-inch pie pan and place the mixture onto it. Now it is time to make the cream.

Mix the coconut water, sea salt, coconut nectar, vanilla and dried coconut in the food processor until smooth. Then add the coconut butter and process for 1 minute. Let's make the filling now.

Pour the cream in 2 bowls. Whisk the Matcha in one of them and fold the coconut into it. Pour this filling over the crust and keep in the freezer to for 1 hour. Then keep the other bowl in the freezer for 45 minutes and wait till it achieves the consistency of whipped cream.

When both the cream and the filling have achieved the desired consistency, use the cream to top the filling and sprinkle a little bit of Matcha over it. Add a large coconut flake and serve!

MATCHA SMOOTHIE BOWL

What if you could eat a smoothie? Well, this is a recipe that lets you enjoy your smoothie with a spoon, not a straw.

Ingredients

To Make the Smoothie:

Ripe banana, 1, frozen

Almond butter, 1 tablespoon

Teaologists organic culinary Matcha, 1 teaspoon

Spinach, 1 cup

Coconut milk, half a cup (can be replaced with unsweetened almond milk if coconut milk is not available)

Pineapple, ½ (diced and ideally frozen)

Coconut butter, 1 tablespoon (optional)

For the Toppings:

Sliced strawberries, 3

Sliced kiwi 1

Chia seeds, 1 teaspoon

Granola, 1 tablespoon

How to Make

Add all the smoothie ingredients to a blender. Add them one by one as they are listed above. Blend until smooth.

If you want to make it extra creamy, you can add a little bit of Greek yoghurt and sugar as desired. Your smoothie is ready! Just take a spoon and dive in!

9 The Future of Matcha

This green tea with a 900-year old history in Japan, is now popular across the world and for good reason. Serve it hot in a bowl (*chawan*), make a latte with it, blend it in a chilled beverage such as iced tea, or cook with it. Matcha is as versatile as it comes.

In modern-day Japan, Matcha is added to everything from Kit Kats to ice creams. Everybody loves Matcha in Japan and enjoy it on a regular basis.

Outside Japan, Matcha is now served at some Starbucks and coffee shops. Matcha desserts are served at restaurants. Companies like Twitter, Evernote, and Airbnb have made Matcha tea available to their employees because of its productivity-boosting, alertness-boosting and concentration-boosting properties.

Matcha is being enjoyed at the office, at home, at the gym, at the coffee shop, and on the commute. As more of its health giving benefits are researched, understood and shared, more people across the world are turning to Match tea and making it part of their daily diet.

Producing good quality Matcha is difficult. Producing great Matcha is, needless to say, even more difficult. It's a labour-intensive and expensive operation. A few companies in Taiwan and China are trying to produce Matcha on a larger scale but the results in both its taste and health giving properties are at best mixed.

Few have the knowledge to produce good Matcha, which is another reason for its limited production.

We all want to live long and healthy lives but we don't always eat and exercise in as disciplined a way as we ought. Matcha tea, with its renowned health-giving properties, can support us in our best efforts to stay fit and well, and help compensate when we occasionally let our disciplines slip.

Teaologists are committed to bringing you the best Matcha tea available, full of flavour and full of all those amazing health benefits. We want you to feel energised, alert and in a good mood every day, ready to achieve your potential with the help of your daily morning Matcha.

10 Matcha Teaware

To fully enjoy Matcha, you need the right tools. What are those tools, you ask? Well, here's everything you need to know about Matcha teaware (a.k.a the tools).

Chawan (Matcha Bowl)

We wouldn't drink fine wine from a tumbler, and likewise, we shouldn't drink Matcha tea from a mug. Well, maybe you can drink it from a mug, but that's definitely not where you prepare it.

The chawan is a utensil that has been used to prepare Matcha tea for 800-900 years. Not only does it serve the purpose of being a vessel that you drink your Matcha from, but it also is a thing of beauty and art that is to be appreciated.

Matcha bowls come in a variety of sizes and shapes from 12.2 cm (4.8 inches) to 15.2 cm (8.98 inches). Remember, if you can't move the whisk well, you need to use a different bowl because the Matcha will be lumpy and not delicious at all. To move the bamboo whisk, the Matcha bowls have to be of a particular size. So naturally, they are much larger than teacups.

Chasen (Bamboo Whisk)

In a never-used bamboo whisk, the bristle tips are well-curved. But after a few uses, they uncurl. Usually made by hand-splitting from only one piece of bamboo, the chasen is susceptible to dry weather conditions. If kept in dry conditions for some time, a hairline crack can develop on the handle of the bamboo whisk It's natural for bamboo to crack in dry weather and will not affect the usability of the whisk. Simply wet the whisk with water before using.' However, even with a crack along the handle, there are no differences in the whisk's usability. Teaologists recommends that you use the whisk for as long as it lasts.

However, if you live in a very dry region, simply wet the entire whisk frequently, and definitely before whisking a bowl of Matcha. This will prevent breakage, as the bristles of the whisk become stronger and more flexible with water.

The bamboo whisk stays neat when kept on a holder.

Chashaku (Matcha Scoop)

Made out of good quality bamboo, the chashaku looks more like a spatula, even though it's used as a scoop. It has a shape that's ideal for measuring Matcha as well as pushing it through the sieve. It is actually the most authentic way to measure Matcha tea before brewing. One small scoop is usually around 1 gram, which is perfect for 1 bowl of Matcha.

Matcha Sieve

Why do you need to sieve Matcha? Because Matcha is so finely ground, when it comes in contact with the static electricity in the air, it becomes lumpy. So if you don't sieve your Matcha, the drink will become lumpy and ruin the drinking pleasure. The sieve makes a perfect Matcha which is smooth to drink. Unlike the other Matcha tools, you don't need to wash the sieve. Instead, simply dust it with a clean toothbrush.

A set of quality Match tools is an asset to your kitchen and to your healthy lifestyle.

11 Disclaimers

All the information in this book is accurate to the best of our knowledge, but please check out the latest research on Matcha tea for yourself.

Matcha tea has many health benefits but please see your doctor if you have any concerns at all or feel unwell. Continue to take any medication as prescribed by your doctor.

Teaologists recommend drinking Matcha in moderation if you are pregnant or nursing. This is due to the caffeine content. A daily intake of 200 mg caffeine is recommended to pregnant women. One cup of Matcha usually contains about 30 mg of caffeine. Please consult your physician before starting to drink Matcha tea on a regular basis.

51702671R00036

Made in the USA
Charleston, SC
01 February 2016